The M Healing _ Honey Every Home Must Have

A DIY Self-Guided Approach to Using Honey Recipes to Heal Over 30 Health Diseases and Infections + Best Tips to Choosing Original Honey

Green Wood

Copyright© 2020 by Green Wood

All right reserved

No part of this publication should be reprinted, stored in a retrieval system, or transmitted in any form or by whatever means, electronic, mechanical, photocopying, recording, or otherwise without the prior consent of the copyright owner.

Acknowledgment

My immense gratitude goes to my research partner, Mr. Oluwafemi Oyenekan, for his massive input in helping put this piece together; his indigenous knowledge of organic herbs formulation is remarkable.

Dedication

I dedicate this book to Almighty God for adding sweetness to our lives and exposing us to the health benefits of honey.

Table of Contents

Acknowledgment iii

Dedication iv

Table of Contents v

Introduction 2

Detecting an Adulterated Honey: How to Identify Pure Original Honey (Procedural Test) 7

The Description of Honey 13

   What is Honey? 13

      The biological process of honey production from honeybees 14

      What does your honey contain? 15

30 Functions and Benefits of Using Pure Original Honey 19

The Curative Power of Pure Original Honey: Recipes, Preparation and Administration . 24

Biblical References of Honey 42

About the Author 45

Author's Contact 46

Introduction

Solomon said, "My son, eat honey, for it is good: the droppings of the honeycomb, which are sweet to your taste" (Proverbs 24:13)

In the Qur'an, Prophet Muhammad strongly advocates the use of honey for therapeutic and healing purposes. This can be found in the book of hadith (al-Nahl), meaning the chapter of the Honey Bee.

Bee therapy, otherwise known as Apitherapy, is a branch of alternative medicine that involves the use of conventional honeybee products for therapeutic purposes. There are biblical events that emphasize the importance of honey. Aside from its sweetness, traditional health practitioners have regarded the healing power of honey in high esteem. During World War I (1914-1918), honey was used on the battlefield as a quick treatment for wounds.

Before antibiotics drugs became ubiquitous (common and found everywhere), honey was used to treat some form of bacterial infections. However, the introduction of antibiotics has trivialized the efficacy of honey as a curative substance to bacterial infections.

An average teaspoon of honey contains about 25 calories. It can convert rapidly and efficiently into energy, unlike the refined white sugar. In other words, honey is quickly metabolized by the body, and it enters into the bloodstream slowly in contrast to how the refined sugar rushes into the bloodstream pushing the pancreas into undue action and pressure.

You are about to be exposed to the mysterious use of honey as a curative to several infirmities and diseases. The beauty of this exposition is that you can do it all by yourself without having to consult a doctor or health practitioner; they are all-natural easy-to-get recipes. You are on a journey of life, a journey of purpose in the quest to identify the natural cure and prevention to those unbearable diseases and life-threatening infirmities all by yourself using honey and some other health benefitting herbal products.

Please take your time, relax, learn, and explore the information adequately as instructed.

Disclaimer

Please be informed that the author is not guaranteeing you absolute healing from the honey herbal recipes. However, consistent usage has been proven to be effective. However, if you don't feel better or observe any significant improvement after days, you can discontinue the usage of the medication.

<u>Warning</u>

For best results, ensure you purchase pure original bee honey, as it determines the effectiveness of the procedures listed in this book. Buying counterfeit or impure honey could endanger health rather than cure, as it is capable of exposing you to the danger of diabetes.

Detecting an Adulterated Honey: How to Identify Pure Original Honey (Procedural Test)

There are several adulterated kinds of honey in the market these days. It takes more than 'taste' to distinguish between pure honey and a mixed one. When you are purchasing honey, ensure you carry out one or two of these tests at the spot before taking it home. A honey sample that passes the four criteria to be discussed is undoubtedly pure original honey.

1. Water Test

When you put original honey in a transparent cup of water, it is expected that it will go down rather than float. It does not dissolve in water or mix uniformly until you stir it your spoon.

Meanwhile, if it stays afloat on the water surface or mixes with the water before stirring, then it is a good sign that you are dealing with counterfeit or impure honey.

2. Matches Test

Get your matches box, pick out a match-stick, and dip the head of the match-stick into the container of your honey and allow it to get wet. Proceed to strike it.

If it ignites a fire, then it is pure original honey. If it doesn't, then it is unlikely the type of honey you want to keep in your home.

3. Against the ground

Allow a drop of your honey to fall to the ground; if it does not penetrate the ground but instead forms a ball-like shape object or roll-like ball, then it is a likely a pure original honey. On the other hand, if it penetrates the ground or flows in a flat-like manner, then it is unlikely pure original honey.

4. Test with fresh-raw meat

Pure original honey is an excellent preservative, rub it on fresh raw meat and leave it till the next day without refrigerating it. If the meat remains fresh without a foul odor, be sure you have used healthy honey.

Beware of unhealthy honey

Test Summary

Test	A pure original honey	An unhealthy honey
1. Put your honey in a transparent cup of water.	The honey will go down to the bottom of the cup, and not mix except when stirred.	It will float and mix with the water without stirring.
2. Dip the head of your match stick in the honey and attempt to strike it.	It will ignite a fire.	It will not ignite a fire.
3. Drop a little content of your	It forms a ball-like shape and does not	It penetrates the ground.

honey to hit the ground	penetrate the ground immediately.	
4. Use it to preserve raw fresh meat without refrigerating	The meat will remain fresh without foul odor.	The meat starts showing signs of spoilage.

The Description of Honey

Meet the major species of the honey bee in the world:

Western Honey (Apis mellifera)

Giant Honey bee (Apis dorsata)

Eastern Honey bee (Apis cerana)

Little Honey bee (Apis florea)

What is Honey?

Honey is a naturally thick, sweet, supersaturated sugar solution produced by bees. It is produced from the honey sacs of various bees. Pure honey should be dark golden.

Notably, honey is the purest source of natural sugar, as it contains forms of sugar such as glucose and fructose, as well as water, oils, and enzymes (Bear in mind that we are referring to pure honey and not a diluted and counterfeit one). It is a natural alternative to white sugar.

The biological process of honey production from honeybees

The process begins with the bees feeding on flowers, and hence collecting the flower nectar in their mouth. In an alchemical process, the nectar mixes with special enzymes in the bee's saliva, which turns to honey. The bee takes the honey back to their hive and then deposits it into the cells of the hive's walls. (You can read more on this if you are interested in bee farming).

Honey bees are the main pollinator of many edible plants; without them, many plant species would have gone into extinction due to lack of pollinating agents.

What does your honey contain?

It has been scientifically proven that natural honey is primarily composed of carbohydrates (in various forms) and water and also contains a trace amount of a wide range of vitamins and minerals.

The nutritional compositions are given in the tabular form:

Minerals	**Vitamins**
Sodium (Na)	Thiamine (B1)
Calcium (Ca)	Riboflavin (B2)
Potassium (K)	Niacin (B3)
Magnesium (Mg)	Pantothenic acid (B5)
Phosphorus (P)	Pyridoxine (B6)
Iron (Fe)	Folic acid (B9)
Copper (Cu)	Ascorbic acid (C)
Manganese (Mn)	Phyllochinon (K)

However, human error or mismanagement or inimical practices can make honey to contain some heavy and toxic metals such as Cadmium (Cd), Lead (Pb), Arsenic (As), and some others.

In addition, honey has some peculiar characteristics that make them an effective curative substance to several ailments. Below are some of the properties of honey that makes them useful in alternative medicine:

Honey has bactericidal, expectorant, and allergenic anti-inflammatory properties, which enhances the body's immuno-biological defense against foreign harmful substances.

Honey possesses an antioxidants property that helps to fight against toxic substances in the bloodstream, hence helping prevent harmful infections.

Honey has a remarkable healing property due to the anti-bacterial agent (Hydrogen peroxide) found in all honey.

30 Functions and Benefits of Using Pure Original Honey

According to scientific research and evidence, regular consumption of honeybee products has proven to help you achieve the following potential health benefits:

1. Improves weak or strained eyes
2. Treats malnutrition especially in kids
3. Improves mental alertness and balance
4. It enhances anabolic support

5. It treats liver ailments and disorder
6. Prevents and treats bladder infections
7. Prevents and treats ulcers
8. Reduces symptoms of eczema
9. Prevents hair loss
10. Relieves heartburn
11. It alleviates prostate discomfort
12. Relieves symptoms of skin disease such as impetigo
13. It alleviates insomnia (sleeplessness)
14. It prevents and cures asthma attack
15. It provides anabolic support
16. It corrects hormonal imbalances especially in females

17. It protects and reduces the risk of coronary artery disease
18. It helps to trivialize menopause-related symptoms
19. Promotes wound healing
20. It helps to treat and correct bladder infections
21. It helps to reduce high blood pressure
22. Helps to reduce cholesterol and blood lipids
23. Helps in tissue and muscle building
24. It helps fight against respiratory infections
25. It promotes healthy, smooth and toned skin
26. It is an anti-aging agent

27. It combats chronic fatigue
28. It stimulates memory and mental function
29. It reduces the extreme craving for food
30. It strengthens the immune system to fight against bacterial and viral infections.

Note: The benefits of honey are not limited to the list above.

> **Notice**
>
> *The Honey Medical Recipes to be discussed below can be used together with other medications serving the same purpose. Most of the recipes works more effectively as preventive measures; therefore, don't wait till the situation is critical before you spring into action.*

The Curative Power of Pure Original Honey: Recipes, Preparation and Administration

> ### __Warning__
>
> For best results, ensure you purchase pure original bee honey, as it determines the effectiveness of the procedures listed in this book.

1. Stooling

Recipes: Onion and pure honey

Preparation: Grind a medium-sized onion and mix with pure honey

Administration: Take two spoonful thrice daily

Note: After the first day, the stooling should subside significantly.

2. Stomach Ulcer/Heartburn

Recipes: Unripe plantain and pure honey

Preparation: Take off the back of the unripe plantain; dry it so that it can be ground into powder.

Administration: Take a teaspoon of the powdery unripe plantain and mix it with 1-2 teaspoons of honey.

3. Irritant Cough

Recipes: Bitter kola (3 pieces), lime (2 pieces), and honey

Preparation: Grind the bitter kola, squeeze the lime, take out about 250ml of honey, and mix it with the grinded bitter kola and the squeezed lime.

Administration: Take a teaspoonful of the mixture thrice a day.

4. High Blood Pressure

Recipes: Ginger, Garlic, lime (optional), and honey.

Preparation: Grind (pound) the ginger and the garlic together to extract the juice, you can add a little quantity of lime juice; mix the mixture with honey (about half of the ginger-garlic mixture).

Administration: Use a tablespoon twice a day (Morning and night).

5. Asthma cough

Recipes: White onion (used in making salad) and honey

Preparation: Grind the white onion, mix with the honey

Administration: Take a tablespoon thrice daily.

6. Insomnia/Sleeplessness

Recipes: Milk and honey

Preparation: Prepare milk using warm water; add two (2)

teaspoons of honey to the warm milk.

Administration: Drink the before going to bed.

7. Arthritis

Recipes: Pear seed (Avocado pear), and honey

Preparation: Dry the seed and grind it into powder, and then mix with the honey.

Administration: Rub on the affected parts.

8. For pile

Recipes: Aloe vera gel and honey

Preparation: Extract the aloe vera gel, and then mix with natural honey.

Administration: Take a tablespoon early in the morning.

9. Rheumatism

Recipes: Garlic and honey

Preparation: Grind the garlic to extract the juice, and then mix with your honey.

Administration: Take one tablespoon daily.

10. Sore throat

Recipes: Lemon juice, salt, and honey

Preparation: Mix two tablespoons of honey with four tablespoons of the lemon juice and add a pinch of salt.

Administration: Gargle the mixture about thrice daily until you feel relieved.

11. Diabetes

Recipes: Mistletoe leaf, aloe vera gel, and honey

Preparation: dry the mistletoe leaf, when dried, boil it until the water turns into a tea-like liquid. Add aloe vera gel along with honey.

Administration: Take half of a glass cup for up to 5 weeks.

12. Bodyweight regulation

Recipes: Lemon and honey

Preparation: Extract the lemon juice and mix it with honey.

Administration: Take out two tablespoons of the lemon juice and mix with three tablespoons of honey. Take the mixture every morning before breakfast, and continue until you get a desirable result.

13. Hair loss/breaking of hair

Recipes: Aloe vera gel and honey

Preparation: Mix the aloe vera gel with the honey.

Administration: Message on the hair scalp and leave it for about 30 minutes before washing it off.

14. Loss of voice/cracked voice

Recipes: Bitter kola (3 pieces), lime (2 pieces), and honey

Preparation: Grind the bitter kola, squeeze the lime, take out about 250ml of honey, and mix it with the grinded bitter kola and the squeezed lime.

Administration: Take a teaspoonful of the mixture thrice a day.

15. Vomiting

Recipes: Pap (Custard; or any semi-liquid food), lime, bitter leaf juice, and honey

Preparation: Prepare the pap, while hot, add a little lime and bitter-leaf juice, and then add honey.

Administration: It should be taken once.

16. Poor erection in man

Honey enhances proper erection in man. If you want to use honey as a remedy for weak erection, use a tablespoon of honey dissolved in half glass of hot water an hour or thirty minutes before sex.

17. Hangover control

Honey is a mixture can speed up the oxidation of alcohol by the liver. You can take about 2-3 tablespoonful of honey when you experience a hangover from drinking too much alcohol.

18. Reddish eyes ball/ Mucus strands in the eyes

Add two tablespoons of pure honey to a cup of boiled water, allow it to cool (lukewarm), use it to rinse the eyes twice daily.

19. Dry skin

Mix honey with shea butter or any cream of your choice. It can be rubbed on your body 10-15 minutes before bathing.

20. Blood lipids and cholesterol

Instead of using the regular white refined sugar, you can use honey as a substitute for sugar in your tea and other liquid or semi-liquid food that requires sugar. The antioxidant nature of honey makes it fight against cholesterol and has the potential to combat heart diseases.

21. Anti-cancer

Honey is not a cure for cancer; however, it has carcinogenic preventing and anti-tumor properties.

22. A bed-wetting kid

If you have a kid that is still bedwetting, give two tablespoons of honey to the kid before going to bed.

23. For wound healing, burns, and cuts

Clean the wound surfaces with an antiseptic liquid and then apply honey directly on the surface of the wound using cotton wool.

24. Measles

Add honey to the juice extract of bitter leaf vegetable. Rub the solution on the affected part. Take a teaspoon (children) and one tablespoon for adults.

25. Eczema

Extract the juice from bitter leaf plant, and then add aloe vera. Mix with honey, and then rub on the affected area.

26. Rashes from after-shave

To prevent rashes from after-shave, you can rub honey on the part you shave to keep the skin part of the area smooth.

27. Ear-aches or any form of pain in the ear

Drop into the affected ear two drops of honey, and then use cotton wool to cover the ear. This is much effective when you do it at night.

28. Loss of appetite

Losing your appetite can be resolved using a mixture of grape juice and honey.

29. Energy booster

Honey is a natural energy booster. It supplies glucose to the body, which is quickly absorbed by the body to give an instant energy boost. If you are on a low feed, take a spoon of honey to keep you sustained for some minutes to a few hours.

30. Immune booster

Taking honey with warm water and lemon juice can be very beneficial in helping build one's immune system. Honey, on its own, is a powerful immune system booster. A spoonful of the mixture daily can be of great advantage.

Biblical References of Honey

My son, eat honey, for it is good: the droppings of the honeycomb, which are sweet to your taste (Proverbs 24:13)

...therefore he put forth the end of the rod who was in his hand, and dipped it in the <u>honeycomb</u>, and put his hand to his mouth;<u> his eyes were enlightened.</u> (1 Samuel 14:27b)

"Then Jonathan said, "My father has troubled the land. Please look how my <u>eyes have been enlightened, because I tasted a</u>

little of this honey. (1 Samuel 14:29)

And he has brought us into this place, and has given us this land, a land flowing with milk and honey (Deuteronomy 26:9)

The house of Israel called its name Manna, and it was like coriander seed, white; and its taste was like wafers with honey. (Exodus 16:31)

He shall eat butter and honey when he knows to refuse the evil, and choose the good. (Isaiah 7:15)

John was clothed with camel's hair and a leather belt around his waist.

He ate locusts and wild honey. (Mark 1:6)

Pleasant words are a honeycomb, sweet to the soul, and health to the bones. (Proverbs 16:24)

I took the little book out of the angel's hand, and ate it up. It was as sweet as honey in my mouth. When I had eaten it, my stomach was made bitter. (Revelation 10:10)

About the Author

Green Wood (Pen name) is a seasoned writer who focuses on herbal products and their health benefits.

His journey through some parts of the west and east Africa and Asia in search of herbal products and their health benefits stresses his passion for the application of natural organic products and their health benefits.

He has constantly been in search of natural cure and prevention to various health deficiencies.

Author's Contact

Contact the author via his email: greenwoodherbalhealth@gmail.com

He is open to questions, inquiries and suggestions.

Printed in Great Britain
by Amazon